Thyme & Oregano

Healing and Cooking Herbs, and more than 30 ways to use them

More books by Evelyn Key:

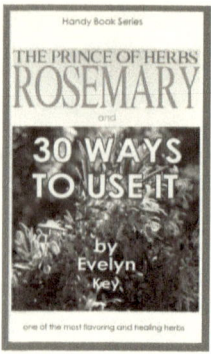
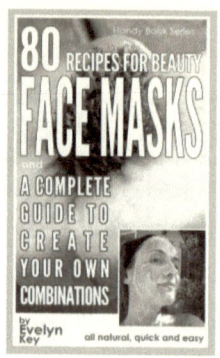

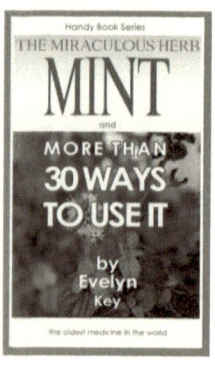
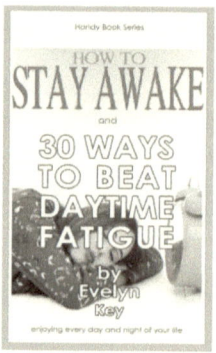

Thyme & Oregano
Healing and Cooking Herbs and more than 30 ways to use them

Evelyn Key

Handy Book Series
2014

First Printing: 2014

ISBN 978-1-312-66218-6

Evangelia Karageorge
P.O. 1866, Agios Spyridon, Porto Rafti
Markopoulo, Attica, Greece, 19003

Handy Book Series
evelinbooks.wordpress.com
evelynbooks@gmail.com

Dedication

To all the optimist, happy and devoted people of this planet!

You create your life, you create the world!

Contents

Introduction

Thyme and Oregano: two of the most famous Mediterranean herbs!

Even though I'm following the same spirit of the series previous books, I'm still trying to improve each new book by making a few changes or additions.

The most obvious difference, is that this book presents two herbs instead of one. If I tried to find a reason why I chose thyme and oregano in the first place, I would say that these two fit together somehow, probably because of their scent and quality, which is actually true in chemical terms because they both contain phenols thymol and carvacrol.

[Today, the species Coridothymus Capitatus is traded as "oregano", because the common feature: their smell, due to the presence of carvacrol in both thyme and oregano essential oils.]

These two wonderful herbs are quite famous as cooking flavourings but also for their superb healing properties.

So, let's see some general info about each one of them.

THYME – The "killing" scent

Thyme is well known as the plant with the most pharmaceutical and therapeutic properties. It was established as a medicine in the 16th century.

Besides the wild thyme, there are over 100 varieties derived from it. Thyme belongs to the family of Labiatae and classified Tubiflorae. The Thymus genus includes about 300 species and many hybrids.

Lemon thyme (Thymus Citriodorus) has larger leaves than the common thyme, and it is a wild thyme variety (T. Serpyllum), very durable with strong aroma.

Cultivate and Collect: Thyme is a low and perennial shrub that doesn't exceed 1.5 feet in height, very durable with small purple flowers. It grows in dry and infertile fields, as well as on mountain slopes, but it can also be grown in the garden as an ornamental plant.

Thyme is propagated by seeds, cuttings and suckers. It can be found in southern and Mediterranean regions of Europe, also in various parts of Asia, while it is cultivated in North America.

Place the thyme pot in a sunny spot, as outside your kitchen window; bellow, you will find several ways to use it in your cooking recipes! Its flavour is quite strong and slightly acrid.

Thyme doesn't need much watering; in fact, it can rot by excessive watering. You can let it outdoors during the winter months, as it is quite resistant to low temperatures.

It blooms from May to early autumn. The useful parts of the plant are the leaves and the flowering tops. Collect them from June to August, during the dry and sunny days. Hang bunches of thyme, upside down and covered with a tulle cloth, in a shaded area and allow to dry. Store it dried in glass jars, or just cut sprigs with leaves and flowers and use them fresh as they are. Thyme should be dried at temperatures below 105°F in order to maintain its flavour and colour.

All kinds of thyme are proper for apiculture, while the essential oil is used in perfumery and cosmetics.

Thyme around the world and through time: Thyme name comes from the ancient Greek word "THYO" (theo) which means something like "offering to the Gods, under the incense smoke." However, according to another aspect, "Thyme" comes from the Greek word "Thymon" which means courageous. Also, the original meaning of the word "Thymos" was "vital force", not anger, as it is nowadays.

In ancient Greece thyme was burned as an offering to the gods, and according to a legend, it was born from the tears of the Beautiful Helen (Helen of Troy). Since the time of Homer, thyme has been a symbol of strength and bravery.

Roman soldiers used it to become stronger and vigorous, the Egyptians for its aromatic qualities and also in the mummification process, while the Sumerians, used thyme 5500 years ago as a spice and also as medicine.

It contains: Tannins, phenols Thymol and Carvacrol, terpinene, cymene, cumin, linalool. The main component of the thyme essential oil is thymol (also called thyme camphor) at 20-54%.

Finally, we shouldn't forget the exceptional quality "thyme honey" with the famous delicious aroma and taste, and its highly beneficial properties.

OREGANO – The queen of aromatic herbs

Although the pharmaceutical companies are not interested in it because it is very cheap, Oregano is an excellent medicine herb.

Oregano belongs to the Lamiaceae family and the Origanum genus. There are four different kinds of oregano, and the most common in Greece is "Oreganum vulgare spp. hirtum. Coridothymus Capitatus is the Spanish, and Origanum Onites the Turkish oregano.

The largest crops are located in Greece and Germany.

The quality of oregano is largely determined by the constituent carvacrol, which is found in oregano oil and ranges from 70 to 85%.

The Greek oregano essential oil is considered the best in the world because, according to credentials, it has a high content in Carvacrol (78,5) while the Thymol content is low (3,9).

Cultivate and Collect: Oregano is drought-resistant, and requires a well-drained soil. Blooms from May to September, and the flowers are white to pink-blue.

Easy to cultivate, it thrives in mountains, fields and gardens. If you have a balcony or at least a sunny kitchen window, you should definitely have an oregano pot!

Oregano is is propagated either by seeds or cuttings. The planting should be done in the period from October to late spring. It doesn't need much watering, in fact, excessive watering degrades the quality of oregano.

Collect sprigs for drying when yellow leaves appear at the base of the plant. However, you can cut and use sprigs of oregano throughout the year. Cut a few, rinse and dry on absorbent towel, and then, tie them in bunches. Hang the bunches, covered with a tulle, in a shady place until the leaves get dried. Then, use a strainer (not too thin), place it over a large bowl, and rub the oregano in it, so the small grated leaves fall into the bowl. Store the grated oregano in a glass jar.

Thyme & Oregano – Healing and Cooking Herbs

Oregano around the world and time: Its name comes from the Greek words "Oros", which means mountain, and "Ganos" which means brightness:

"The plant that brightens the mountains"

According to Greek mythology, Aphrodite created oregano to make people's lives happier. In ancient times, the newlyweds were crowned with garlands of oregano to have a happy life, while it was cultivated even close to the tombs, to offer peace and tranquility to the spirits of the dead.

Greeks and Egyptians used oregano mostly as a preservative, as an antidote to poisons, and as a remedy for skin diseases and infections.

In the Middle Ages people chewed oregano leaves for indigestion, rheumatism, toothache and coughs.

The British used to smoke oregano. In America, oregano became known after the Second World War, when the American soldiers learned and loved this herb after their invasion in Italy in 1943.

It contains: The phenolic compounds carvacrol and thymol. It is a source of vitamins C, K and A, and also contains pinene, ursolic, caffeic and rosmarinic acid, iron, beta-carotene and fibre

Thyme and Oregano have always been two of the main medicinal herbs, the "guards of health", and they weren't missing from any Greek house of the past.

Please check on cautions and always keep them in mind. Thank you!

Cautions

Thyme:
- Over consumption (or daily internal use) can cause an overactive thyroid gland, poisoning, vomiting, diarrhoea, dizziness, depression. Do not to drink much and for long periods. In cases of colds or other treatment, consumption of 2-3 cups a day cannot exceed 1 week period.
- It is not recommended for use by hypertensive people because it elevates blood pressure.
- Do not use during pregnancy because thyme is a uterine stimulant.

Oregano:
- Should be avoided by pregnant women and people who suffer from iron deficiency.
- Avoid the use of essential oil in children under 4 years

General cautions:
- If you take any medication, always consult your therapist before you use herbal treatments, because some herbs may be inappropriate in your condition or it might eliminate/increase the action of your medications.
- Never use essential oils directly to your skin; never consume them undissolved.

■

"Each day is a little life: every waking and rising a little birth, every fresh morning a little youth, every going to rest and sleep a little death."
Arthur Schopenhauer

"Laugh and the world laughs with you, snore and you sleep alone."
Anthony Burgess

"Think in the morning. Act in the noon. Eat in the evening. Sleep in the night."
William Blake

"A well-spent day brings happy sleep."
Leonardo Da Vinci

Heal and Protect

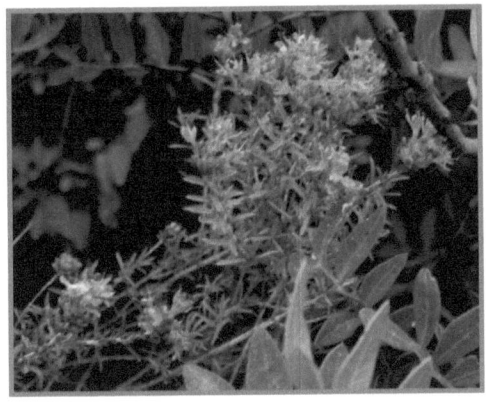

The inhalation of **oregano** substances helps with lung problems such as bronchitis, asthma, etc.

Studies of the Aristotle University of Thessaloniki, showed that **oregano** acts effectively for lowering blood sugar, while it has antioxidant activity.

The healing properties of **thyme** have been known since the time of Hippocrates.

Colds and Flue
THYME

Thyme is a preventive antibiotic for flu epidemics. Hippocrates, in his writings on Diet, says the **thyme** is heating, diuretic and expels phlegm. **Thyme** heals bronchitis and strengthens the immune system against the flu or colds.

- Drink a thyme infusion 3 times a day, for 3 days in a row (never exceed a week period).
- Drink half a glass of lukewarm water with 5 drops of thyme tincture (or 1 drop of thyme essential oil), 3 times a day, for 3 days in a row (after meals) [**Note:** The thyme essential oil can act as a_febrifuge because it causes profuse sweating, so it helps the blood toxin removal.]
- Rub your chest and your back with your homemade thyme tincture or oil extract.
- Do steam inhalations over hot infusion of thyme. Alternatively, in a bowl with hot water, add 8 drops of thyme essential oil and inhale the steam.
- Prepare a thyme beeswax salve, and rub your chest and neck with it.

- Six drops of thyme essential oil mixed with three teaspoons of almond oil for chest rubs; helps with lung infections.

OREGANO

Oregano strengthens the respiratory and immune system.
"If you want to sneeze, rub your nose with **oregano.**"

- For nasal decongestion: Drip three drops of oregano essential oil on a handkerchief, and put it on your pillow at night, to inhale the scent. Or inhale the steam over a hot oregano infusion.
- For colds and runny nose: Gargle with cool decoction of oregano.
- For colds: Drink a glass of water or orange juice with 2 drops of oregano essential oil or 5 drops of oregano tincture (noon and evening.)
- For fever: drink a hot infusion of oregano with cinnamon.

Related issues:

".. *Thyme (*Thymus vulgaris*) -- Thyme has traditionally been used to treat respiratory illnesses such as bronchitis and to treat cough. Two preliminary studies suggest that thyme may help treat acute bronchitis and relieve cough. Thyme is approved by the German Commission E to treat those conditions. Thyme oil is considered toxic and should not be taken by mouth. Thyme may increase the risk of bleeding, especially if you also take blood-thinners such as aspirin, clopidogrel (Plavix), or warfarin (Coumadin)...* [Cough | University of Maryland Medical Center]

Cough
THYME

The moment you feel the first tickle in your throat, try some thyme. It has a preventive effect.

- In cases of cough or whooping cough, try a spoonful of honey mixed with 1 drop of thyme essential oil and 1 of eucalyptus, for a 3-4 days (morning, noon and evening).
- The thyme decoction or infusion can also treat coughs and bronchitis. Combine with mint and sage. Add 1 tsp honey
- **Cough Syrup recipe**
  Ingredients:
  1 ounce dry thyme

8 ounces brown sugar
8 ounces honey
2 cups of distilled water
Preparation: Put the dry thyme in a ceramic pot and pour the boiling water. Let it stay for about 15 minutes in order to absorb all the beneficial substances. Strain into another pot and place it over low heat. Add the sugar and the honey and stir continuously. Skim when it starts to boil. When it starts to thicken, remove from fire and let it cool. Store it in the fridge in a dark glass bottle with a cork.

Usage: 1 tbsp, morning and night. Do not take it longer than a week. See cautions.

- **An easier and lighter syrup recipe**
Boil 2 cups of water with 2 cups of thyme until the 1/3 of the water evaporates. Then remove from the fire, cover and let stand for 5-10 minutes. Strain, add 4 tbsp honey and mix well. Put in a small glass bottle.

Usage: 3 tbsp a day after meals (morning-noon-night and a maximum of one week). Store in the fridge and shake before use.

OREGANO

- Decoction of oregano, made with a teaspoon of dry oregano for each cup of water. Add 1 tsp honey and drink hot; ½ cup, 3 times a day.
- Mix 1 tablespoon oregano with 1 cup of honey. Eat a spoonful of the mixture 3 times a day. (This practical advice comes from Ioannina, Greece)

Related issues:
"Oral treatment of acute bronchitis with thyme-primrose combination for about 11 days was superior to placebo in terms of efficacy. The treatment was safe and well tolerated." [German study] [1]

Diarrhoea
While you suffer from diarrhoea, try to avoid drinking coffee, milk and alcohol or eating spicy and fatty foods. And try these two herbs which can be actually very beneficial.

THYME

Because of its mild astringent action, thyme is useful in child-hood diarrhoea and bed wetting.

- For diarrhoea that comes from cold belly, 5 drops of thyme tincture in half a glass of water, 3 times a day.
- Drink an infusion three times a day, for three days.

OREGANO

Oregano helps diarrhoea because it has spasmolytic, antimicrobial and antidiarrheal properties.

- Drink ½ cup of oregano decoction 2-3 times a day, before meals; no honey or sugar. It doesn't taste so good, but it is a medicine after all! You can prepare it in the morning and drink it during the day.
- As a second option: while you make the oregano decoction, add ½ lemon (whole, not just the juice) and let it boil with the oregano. Drink as above.

Related issues:

".. *Oil of Mediterranean oregano Oreganum vulgare was orally administered to 14 adult patients whose stools tested positive for enteric parasites, Blastocystis hominis, Entamoeba hartmanni and Endolimax nana. After 6 weeks of supplementation with 600 mg emulsified oil of oregano daily, there was complete disappearance of Entamoeba hartmanni* (four cases), *Endolimax nana* (one case), *and Blastocystis hominis in eight cases. Also, Blastocystis hominis scores declined in three additional cases. Gastrointestinal symptoms improved in seven of the 11 patients who had tested positive for Blastocystis hominis.* [Copyright © 2000 John Wiley & Sons, Ltd.] (2)

"*Research has shown that thyme essential oil can decontaminate Shigella on lettuce. Shigella sonnei is a bacteria that causes diarrhoea. Washing vegetables and fruits with just 1 per cent of thyme essential oil added to the wash, dropped the number of Shigella bacteria below the detection point.*" [Greenchedy](3)

Disinfectant

THYME

Thyme's antibacterial properties, have been shown by experiments conducted in 1887 by Chamberland[4], later by Candeac and Meunier (1889) and many others. Thyme essential oil is 25 times more antiseptic than hydrogen peroxide.

For the ancient Greeks, thyme was the number one disinfectant, and also, a symbol of courage.

- Eight drops of thyme tincture in a glass of distilled water can be used for gargling for oral or throat problems.
- Use the thyme tincture as a hand sanitizer.
- Burn dry thyme as an incense to disinfect the air (or use essential oil and an essential oil warmer/diffuser.)
- Add a few drops of essential oil, or thyme oil extract, or thyme tincture, in your bath water for a disinfectant bath, that will also give you strength and courage!
- Clean and disinfect your home and your shoes!
- Disinfect wounds and stings

OREGANO

You can use oregano instead of thyme (or both) in all the above solutions. Oregano has also antimicrobial and antibacterial properties.

Related issues:

"This study was carried out to determine whether oregano (Origanum onites) essential oil works as a disinfectant for hatching egg obtained from broiler breeder flock [..] These results imply that oregano essential oil had great potential for hatching egg disinfectant and it could be used as natural egg disinfectant." [Use of Oregano (Origanum Onites L.) Essential Oil as Hatching Egg Disinfectant]

"..Carvacrol has been found to contain potent anti-fungal and antibacterial properties, with a range of medicinal uses..." (5)

Inappetence
THYME

Thyme stimulates the digestive system and relieves intestinal fermentations. The essential oil of thyme, whets the appetite, relieves abdominal bloating and gas accumulation in the stomach.

- Drink 1 tbsp water with 3 drops of thyme tincture or 1 cup of water with 1 drop of thyme essential oil, half an hour before meals, for 3-4 days.
- Add thyme to your food recipes; its smell can intrigue your appetite as well.
- Prepare and drink a thyme decoction, with 1 tsp thyme, ½ garlic clove, 1tsp lemon, half an hour before meal.

OREGANO

Oregano helps digestion and builds up an appetite.

For a digestive or appetizer solution, add 1 drop of oregano essential oil (or 5 drops of tincture) in a glass of water.

Menstrual problems
THYME

Thyme can help in cases of menstrual cramps and also the PMS symptoms such as pains, headaches etc. The consumption of thyme tea can also help with vaginal infections (yeast infections (candidiasis) or trichomoniasis.)

- Put a compress of thyme over the abdomen. Try to keep it warm; cover the compress with a towel to maintain the warm temperature.
- Massage the abdomen area with warm thyme oil extract and wrap with a warm towel. Wear your clothes above it to maintain the temperature.
- Drink a decoction of thyme flower tops, ½ cup up to 3 times a day, for 2-4 days before or during menstruation.

OREGANO

Oregano is an emmenagogue, so it is appropriate in cases of menstrual irregularity. It also helps during menopause, both in the physical and psychological level.

Drink oregano tea, 2-3 times a day for 5-6 days in case of amenorrhea. Drink ½ cup and remember that even if it doesn't taste so good, it is quite beneficial.

Related issues:
"Various sources have reported that the thyme was recommended for menstrual disorders because of its antispasmodic and astringent effects." (6)

*"Oregano (*Origanum vulgare*) has been used historically to improve circulation as an emmenagogue, for infections of the oral cavity, as a carminative for digestive health, and for the treatment of inflammatory disorders such as arthritis."* (7)

Oral/throat diseases and toothache
Cretans used to rub **thyme** directly on the gums because it fights gum disease.

THYME
The antibacterial properties of thyme can help against oral diseases. Thyme also cleans the teeth, and this is why thymol is commonly used in toothpastes and mouthwashes.

- You can use it to relieve tooth aching until you visit your dentist.
- Sore throat may be caused by several factors, such as viruses, cold, flu or bacteria, allergies, polluted environment, and thyme is one of the most effective bronchial antispasmodics and expectorants.
- Mouthwash: Prepare an infusion of thyme, let it cool down and use it as a mouthwash after meals. **Or** add 1 tsp of thyme tincture into half a glass of water and rinse your mouth. **Or** add 1 drop of thyme essential oil in one cup of water.
- Gargling: You can also use the same formulas as above to gargle. It will improve your mouth hygiene and breath odour.
- Teeth wash: Use a coffee grinder, or a pestle, to turn some dried thyme into a powder. Put the ground thyme in a small glass jar. Take some powder with your toothbrush (no water) and rub it on your teeth. Rinse with water afterwards.

- Toothache: Put a few drops of thyme tincture on a small piece of cotton, place it on the aching tooth, and press your teeth together to keep it there for a while. **Or** Prepare a warm compress and place it on your cheek, where your tooth aches.
- Sore throat: Chewing thyme is effective in cases of sore throat. Its taste is bitter, but highly beneficial.

OREGANO

The infusion of oregano can also be used for mouth washes and gargling. It helps against gingivitis and periodontitis, inflammations and bad breath, while it relieves tooth aching.

- Gingivitis and oral diseases: Mouthwashes and gargling 3 times a day with an infusion of oregano. Also beneficial for sore throat and ulcers.
- Toothache: In a cup of water, add 10 drops of oregano oil extract. Put a portion of the mixture in your mouth and keep it there for a while, close to the tooth that hurts. It acts as a painkiller.

Related issues:

"The essential oils of Oreganum vulgare L. (Oregano) and Thymus vulgaris (thyme) were shown to exhibit a range of biological activities. Both are commonly used in foods, mainly for their flavour, aroma and preservation properties. They were used to delay or inhibit growth of pathogenic microorganisms, as they present strong antimicrobial activity, mostly attributable to the presence of phenolic compounds such as thymol and carvacrol, and to hydrocarbons such as γ-terpinene and p-cymene..." (8)

"Byron Richards, CCN correspondent reported the new findings of an Italian University study, which gives proof of the germ killing properties of oregano oil..." (9)

Rheumatism
THYME

- Six drops of thyme essential oil in 3 tbsp almond or sunflower oil (organic). Rub for rheumatic pains or muscle pullings. (Combine optionally with lavender essential oil)

- Also try thyme baths because they offer wellness, relaxation and relieve pains of rheumatic diseases.

OREGANO

- Massage with oregano oil extract, or oregano essential oil mixed with an organic plant oil such as almond oil. (1 drop of essential oil for each tbsp of almond oil)
- Prepare a beeswax salve with oregano, and rub the suffering areas.
- Here is an oil recipe for rheumatism or muscle crabs and pains.

Ingredients:

4 cups plant oil (almond oil, olive oil, sunflower oil)

3 sprigs of thyme

1 sprig of rosemary

1 handful of lavender

1 handful of sage

½ tsp black pepper

½ tsp red pepper

1 nutmeg

5 cloves

10 dried red hot peppers

1 cinnamon stick

Preparation: Crush all the herbs and spices with a pestle, and then put them in a clean glass jar. Add the oil and close the lid. Place the jar in a shady place and shake once a day. After one month, strain and keep the oil in a dark glass bottle.

You can store it away from high heat and use it for massage suffering muscles and joints.

Skin disorders

THYME

Thyme can treat skin problems such as scabies, lichens and acne. According to researchers[10], thyme tincture can be very effective on skin issues such as acne.

- Prepare a skin lotion: In 3.5Oz Rose water, add 30 drops of thyme tincture and shake well. Apply to a clean face with a cotton pad, every night before you go to bed

- For scabies, lichens, eczema: Mix 1 drop thyme essential oil with 1 tbsp olive oil, and apply to the suffering area 3 times a day. Combine with drinking thyme tea (Note: always be aware of the cautions)
- For scabies: Apply a thyme compress or thyme poultice. These methods can benefit all cases of skin disorders.

OREGANO

Antimicrobial and antiseptic properties of oregano essential oil, help against skin disorders.

- For scabies: Add a decoction of oregano (about 8 cups) to your bath water.
- For acne: Apply a simple, natural face mask. Mix 1 drop of oregano essential oil with 1 tbsp thyme honey. Apply on your skin. Rinse after 15 minutes with lukewarm water and then cold. Repeat up to 2 times a week.

Related issues:

"Researchers from Leeds Metropolitan University tested the effect of thyme, marigold and myrrh tinctures on Propionibacterium ac-nes *-- the bacterium that causes acne by infecting skin pores and forming spots, which range from white heads through to puss-filled cysts. The group found that while all the preparations were able to kill the bacterium after five minutes exposure, thyme was the most effective of the three. What's more, they discovered that thyme tincture had a greater antibacterial effect than standard concentrations of benzoyl peroxide -- the active ingredient in most anti-acne creams or washes. "*[ScienceDaily, source: Society for General microbiology]

Stomach
THYME

Thymol helps the digestion of fatty foods. It also removes intestinal parasites. The anticonvulsant activity of the thyme essential oil, smoothes the muscles, soothes the digestive system and relieves bloating.

- Prepare a thyme infusion. Pour 2 cups of hot water in a pot with 1 tbsp dried thyme. Let it stay for about 10 minutes.

Strain and drink 1 cup after lunch and 1 after dinner. Repeat for 2-3 days if necessary.

- You can add 1 drop of thyme essential oil in your water, after meals, 3 times a day. Do not take for longer than 3-4 days.

OREGANO

Invaluable for stomach problems, particularly in gastric atony. Also very helpful against intestinal disorders and abdominal pains.

- Drink a decoction of oregano 2-3 times a day.
- Add oregano in your salads; it goes perfectly with tomatoes and cucumber, potatoes, beans and more. A stomach medicine in your plate! Try it!
- Drink ½ cup of water with 5 drops of oregano tincture after meals.
- Try oils and vinegars flavoured with thyme and oregano.

Related issues:

"Oil of Mediterranean oregano Oreganum vulgare was orally administered to 14 adult patients whose stools tested positive for enteric parasites, Blastocystis hominis, Entamoeba hartmanni and Endolimax nana. After 6 weeks of supplementation with 600 mg emulsified oil of oregano daily, there was complete disappearance of Entamoeba hartmanni (four cases), Endolimax nana (one case), and Blastocystis hominis in eight cases. Also, Blastocystis hominis scores declined in three additional cases. Gastrointestinal symptoms improved in seven of the 11 patients who had tested positive for Blastocystis hominis." (11)

Stings and bites
THYME

Plinius recommends thyme as an antidote for snake poison, or poisonous bites by sea creatures. The Romans burned thyme to repel scorpions.

- For stings 1 tbsp olive oil and 2 drops of thyme essential oil. Mix and apply on the stung area. **Or** use your homemade thyme oil extract directly on the wounded area; the disinfectant properties will prevent infection.
- Place a cold thyme compress on the suffering area.

OREGANO

According to Aristotle, when a turtle eats a snake, immediately after, eats oregano as a poison antidote.

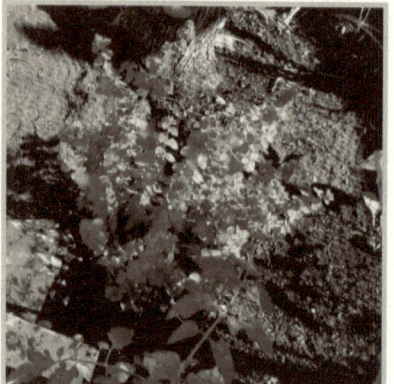

- <u>For bites, and also fungal infections and rashes</u>, mix 2 drops of oregano essential oil with two teaspoons of olive oil. Put the mixture on the suffering area.
- Mix 1 cup apple vinegar with 1 cup oregano infusion or 1 tbsp oregano tincture, and apply compresses of this mixture on the wounded area.
- Stings: apply some beeswax salve.

Stiff neck

THYME

- Compresses of thyme, act against muscle spasms. Make a warm thyme compress.
- Massage with thyme oil extract.
- Apply some thyme beeswax cream and massage.

Oregano:

- Massage with oregano oil extract.
- Prepare a poultice, wrap it within a thin, soft cloth or a gauze, and place it on the hurting area.
- In a dry frying pan, heat some fresh oregano leaves over low fire. Fold them within a soft piece of fabric and place it on the spot that hurts. You can use it also for rheumatism.

Toning

THYME

In ancient Greece, people used to drink an energizing drink made of figs and thyme, simmering in water or wine. I don't have the recipes, but maybe you would like to do your own experiments.

Thyme gives strength, mental clarity, while it helps against mental fatigue and depression.

- <u>Tonic massage</u>: Mix 5 drops of thyme, 3 drops of orange and 2 drops of rosemary essential oils with 3 ounces almond oil, and ask someone to give you a good massage.
- <u>Tonic wine recipe:</u>
  Ingredients:
  4 cups of red wine
  1 tbsp fresh rosemary (not necessarily bloomed)
  1 tbsp fresh mint leaves
  1 tbsp fresh thyme (not necessarily bloomed)
  1 stick cinnamon
  2 ounces of brown sugar

Preparation: Put all herbs in a jar, add the wine, close it well and let the herbs soak for 3 days. Strain and add sugar. Leave it for 15 more days in a dark place. Shake once a day. Drink this stimulating wine in small portions as a liqueur.

Make me Beautiful and Fresh new!

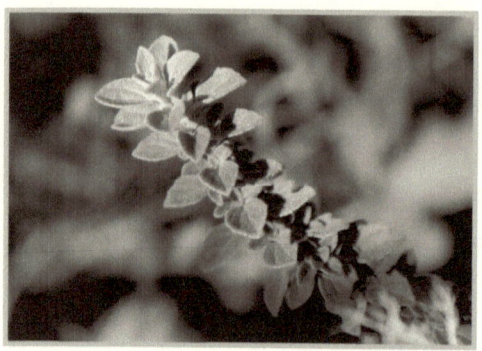

Thyme and oregano offer quite interesting herbal solutions for beauty care and personal hygiene.

Anti-aging

Oregano, due to its antioxidant action and the high content of vitamin C, is one of the finest anti-aging herbs.

OREGANO:

You can use oregano oil extract to moisturize your face, hands and feet, and take advantage of its powerful anti-aging properties.

- Mix 1 drop of oregano essential oil with 1tbsp almond oil and apply on the skin.
- Wash your face with a cool oregano infusion.
- Don't forget to include oregano in your diet.

Body scrubs

THYME:

- **Cellulite scrub**
  You will need:
  ½ cup organic corn oil
  4 tbsp natural grapefruit juice
  1 handful dry thyme flowers and leaves

  How to: Crush the thyme with a pestle. Mix the oil with the juice, and apply on your skin. Let it dry a bit, and then, take some thyme with your fingers and rub your skin gently. Immediately after, enclose the skin area with a piece of plastic wrap and let the heat do the job! After 10-15 minutes, remove the plastic and rinse with luke-warm water first, and then cold.

Thyme cleanses the skin deeply and stimulates blood circulation while grapefruit helps burning fats. Corn oil has anti-aging properties and softens the skin. So, if you combine them, you have a body scrub, ideal for cellulite. Always keep in mind, that the treatment has to be repeated regularly in order to perform actual results,.

- **Next, follows a body scrub for smooth skin, cleansing and protection.**
  You will need:
  1 cup of organic salt
  4 tbsp almond oil (or any organic vegetable oil)
  2 tsp fresh thyme leaves and flowers
  1 lemon or orange zest
  1 clean and dry glass jar with a lid
  How to: Put all the ingredients in the jar and mix well. Take a small portion in your hand and scrub your body, after shower. Then rinse.
  If you have already made some thyme oil extract, you can use it instead of almond oil.

OREGANO:

Black pepper cleans deeply the skin and has also anti-aging properties. Combined with oregano's anti-aging and antiseptic 'skills', makes a 'perfect match' for a cleansing and rejuvenating body scrub!
Anti-aging scrub:
You will need:
2 tbsp black sugar
2 tbsp fine sea salt
1 tbsp ground black pepper
1 tbsp oregano
Any organic plant oil (almond, olive, corn oil)
How to: Mix all the ingredients together. Add as much vegetable oil as needed (about 2-3 tbsp should be enough) and mix well. Take a small portion with your fingers and rub your body gently, in a circular motion. Rinse with lukewarm water.

Cologne
THYME:

This one doesn't have much difference from the tincture formula, however, it is a refreshing and disinfectant cologne:

1 handful of thyme flowers and 1 handful of lavender flowers, 8,5oz white spirit (90% volume). Put them all in a dark glass bottle, close the cap and place it under the sunlight for about 3 weeks; it better be summer season. Smell it and if it is good, strain and use. This cologne is very good for after shaving.

Hair
THYME:

Thyme helps in cases of hair loss. During the ancient times, it was considered an excellent hair tonic.

- Make an infusion of thyme, and massage your scalp after shampooing. Let it stay for about 5-10 minutes and rinse. Repeat on each shampooing for one month.
- Try a hair mask:
You will need:
2 tbsp bay tree oil, 2 drops thyme essential oil, 1 tsp thyme honey. Mix all the ingredients well and apply to dry hair. Let it stay for 30 minutes and wash.

Note: remember to apply the shampoo alone, with no water, because this way is easier to remove the oil from the hair; wash well and then rinse with plenty of water.

OREGANO:

Oregano helps against dandruff and oiliness.

- Solution A:
In a pot, pour 4 cups of water and 1 handful of oregano. Simmer for about 10-15 minutes. Then, strain and put the liquid in a glass bottle.

Before shampooing, massage the scalp with a small portion of the oregano lotion. Apply the treatment for about 20-30 days. Keep the lotion in the refrigerator.

- Solution B:

Pour two cups of boiled water in a pot with 2 teaspoons of dried oregano. Cover and let stand for 6 hours. Strain, add 2 tbsp apple vinegar and mix well.

Store it in a glass bottle. Gently massage your scalp with a small portion of the lotion, let it for half an hour and then wash your hair. Repeat 2-3 times weekly.

Bath salts
THYME:

Relaxing, detoxifying, ideal for puffiness and bruises, for stiff neck, stimulating of blood circulation, immune system boosting, analgesic:

Ingredients:
1 cup Epsom salts
1 cup organic sea salt
2 cups baking soda
5-10 drops of thyme (test to see how strong you want the scent)
Or 2 tbsp thyme oil extract
How to: Mix together and store in a glass jar.
Add Himalayan salts, which are very beneficial for skin disorders such as eczema, scabies, and also great for relaxation, detoxification, muscle issues, and skin improvement.
Use ¼ cup of the salt mixture for each bath.

Caution: Avoid hot baths with salts if you have heart problems or high blood pressure.

Bathing
THYME:

A bath in thyme scented water, provides vitality and vigour. It combats tiredness by offering wellness and relaxation. Also beneficial for arthritis and rheumatism, colds and flu.

- **In your bath water, add one or more of the following:**
  10 drops of thyme essential oil.
  2 tbsp of your homemade thyme oil extract

¼ cup of your homemade bath salts.
- Fold a handful of fresh or dried thyme in a fabric pouch, and toss it into your bath water.
- Make a thyme infusion with 8 cups of water and 1 cup thyme, and mix it with your bath water.

OREGANO:

For a relaxing, stimulating, soothing and rejuvenating bath, add oregano instead of thyme to the above solutions.

Brain tonic

Thyme enhances mental clarity. In ancient Greece, the elderly used to drink infusions of thyme to maintain their mental strength.
- Drink a thyme decoction, 2 cups a day (after meal) for 1 week each month.
- Add 5 drops of thyme tincture in your regular tea. Drink up to 3 times a day, for up to 6-7 days in a row.
- Smell it. Diffuse thyme scent in the air, or have always with you a scented cloth and smell it every time you feel like you need to clear your mind.
- Throw some thyme twigs in the burning fireplace.
- **<u>Wine recipe with thyme and rosemary!</u>**
  Ingredients:
  4 cups red wine
  1 sprig fresh rosemary
  1 ½ tbsp fresh thyme
  5 cloves
  1 ½ -2 ounces brown sugar

Preparation: Put the herbs, the cloves and the sugar in a jar. Pour the wine over them, and close the lid. Let it in a cool and dark place for about ten days. Shake once a day to dissolve the sugar. Then strain, keep it in a dark glass bottle and serve in small glasses as a liqueur.

Smelly feet

One of the most common reasons that cause foot odour, is bacteria. Herbs with antibacterial, antimicrobial, antiseptic and disinfectant properties, can be proven especially useful and effective.

THYME:

- Prepare a strong thyme infusion, with 6 cups of water and 1 ½ cup of thyme leaves and flowers. Soak your feet. Repeat everyday if possible for quicker results.
- Mix 1 cup rose water with 2 drops of thyme essential oil or 1 tbsp thyme tincture. Put it in a spray bottle and spray the feet after shower. Emphasize between the fingers.
- Use the body scrub with thyme and lemon, and enjoy finely cleaned and smooth feet!
- If you wear sneakers, 1 drop of thyme essential oil in each shoe will also help. If your shoes are leather or synthetic, mix 1 tbsp apple vinegar and 1 tbsp thyme tincture and coat the inside of your shoes with a cotton pad. Let dry completely before you wear them.

Let's talk Mediterranean!

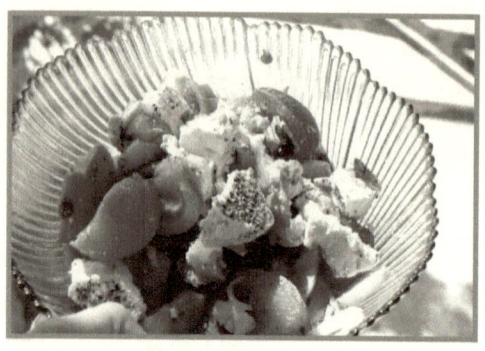

Thyme and oregano are used so often in the Greek/ Mediterranean cuisine, and they both have great taste and aroma! Dried or fresh, their aromatic qualities are exceptional.

There are many ways to try them both and flavour main dishes, marinades, salads, oils, vinegars, sauces and dips, even desserts!

A 1663AC soup recipe with thyme and beer, was well known for its ability to enhance confidence.

Add the herbs at the end of cooking, so to keep their flavour and nutrients.

Marinade

A marinade for grilled vegetables, mushrooms and meat.

Ingredients:

2, ½ cups of white wine

1 bunch of thyme

3 garlic cloves

3 bay leaves

4 cloves.

How to: Cut the garlic cloves into pieces. In a large bowl, pour the wine, add the rest of the ingredients and stir.

Breads (2 recipes)

- **Recipe-1: Cheese bread with thyme**

  Ingredients:

  3 cups of water

  1 tbsp fresh chopped thyme (you can also use dried, but fresh is preferred)

  2 pounds all purpose flour

  2 tsp honey

1 tsp salt
2 sachets of dry yeast
White goat cheese (a little less than 1 pound)
3.5 Oz olive oil
3-4 tsp sesame seeds
Ground pepper

How to: Mix the oil with the honey and the water, and warm the mixture a little bit over low heat (do not overheat or boil). Remove from fire. Pour the mixture in a bowl, add the yeast and stir well until it dissolves.

Put the flour and the salt in a large bowl and mix well. Make a hole in the middle and pour the yeast mixture. Knead to make a soft dough, adding lukewarm water or flour if needed. Cover the bowl with a towel and let it rest in a warm place for half an hour (or until it gets the double of its size)

In another bowl, mash the goat cheese, add the pepper and mix together.

Divide the dough into 6 balls. Use a dough roller to turn each ball into an elongated layer. Put the 1/6 of the cheese along the layer and roll to a cylinder shape. Then shape the stuffed cylinder like a snail shell or like a bagel.

Follow the same procedure with the rest dough and cheese. Cover the breads with a large towel and let them rise again. Sprinkle the sesame seeds and bake at 350F for about 50 minutes.

A snack to enjoy with your beloved ones.

- **Recipe-2:Bread with oregano and thyme**
  Ingredients:
  3 cups of all purpose flour
  1 tsp baking soda
  1 sachet of dry yeast
  ½ cup olive oil
  1 tsp dried thyme
  1 tsp dried oregano
  1 tsp salt
  1 cup lukewarm milk (prefer goat milk)
  Sesame seeds

How to: In a large bowl, add the flour, the herbs, the salt and the baking soda, and mix well. Dissolve the yeast with lukewarm water. Make a hole in the middle of the flour mixture, and pour the yeast, the milk and the olive oil. Mix and knead into a soft and pliable dough; add more milk or flour if needed.

Knead for a few minutes and then shape an oblong loaf. Place it on an oven tray, cover with a towel, and let in a warm place for half an hour to rise a bit. Preheat the oven to 350F.

With the tip of a knife, make 2-3 shallow cuts on the surface of the loaf, sprinkle with sesame seeds, and bake for 50-60 minutes until it gets golden brown.

Eat as an aromatic bread along with your meal, as a snack, or make brouschetta slices.

Pizza

Oregano is a very popular ingredient in pizzas. You can use tomato and oregano almost in every pizza you make!

Ingredients for 2 pizzas
1 pound all purpose flour
1 sachet of dry yeast
1 tbsp oregano
1 tsp sugar
1 tbsp salt
4 tbsp olive oil
Pepper
Warm water

How to: In a cup, dissolve the yeast with lukewarm water (be careful, not too hot because it will ruin the yeast.) In a large bowl, put the flour, the sugar, the salt, the oregano and the pepper and mix them. Pour the dissolved yeast and the olive oil, and knead while adding lukewarm water slowly, until you make a smooth, soft and unified dough. Then cover the bowl with a plastic wrap or just a towel. Put something even warmer above it, like a small blanket, and let it aside to rise (about 1 hour).

Then knead again for a few minutes and divide the dough in two pieces. Spread a few drops of oil at the bottom of two round shape baking pans (about 12inch diameter), and make a layer with each piece of dough with your fingers or with a small dough roller.

Then, add your favourite ingredients on top and bake for about 20 minutes, or store the dough in the freezer for another time.

Potatoes/Eggplants/Peppers

- **Potatoes with thyme and garlic**
  Ingredients:
  2 pounds small round potatoes
  1 cup olive oil
  1 garlic clove
  1 cup fresh thyme leaves and flowers
  Salt, pepper
  How to: Wash the potatoes (don't peel if they are organic) and put them in a baking pan. Chop the garlic. Season the potatoes with salt and pepper, add the oil, the thyme and the garlic, and mix together with your hands. Cover with a tin foil and bake at 300F. Use a toothpick to check if they are ready.
  Combine with marinated roasted vegetables and white wine!

- **Peppers with wine and oregano**
  Ingredients:
  10-15 long and narrow green peppers
  ½ cup olive oil
  ½ cup white wine
  1 tbsp oregano
  Salt and pepper
  How to: Put the oil in a skillet, over low heat, and sauté the peppers whole as they are. Cover and let them for about 5 minutes, until they just wilted. Add the wine, stir a little, cover and let them simmer over low heat for 5-7 more minutes. Season with salt and pepper, add oregano, stir and remove from fire. Serve as an appetizer or with rice.
  You can prepare the same recipe and instead of oregano, garnish with thyme flavoured oil.

- **Eggplants**
  Ingredients
  1 large eggplant
  ½ cup flour

6 tbsp olive oil
3 tbsp thyme honey
2 tbsp thyme leaves
Salt and pepper

How to: Cut a large eggplant into slices and let them soak in salted water overnight. The next day, put the flour on a plate, wring the eggplant slices and put them in the flour on both sides. Heat 3 tbsp of the oil and fry the eggplant slices, to be browned on both sides.

In a bowl, put the honey, the rest of the oil, thyme and a pinch of salt and pepper, and mix well until they unify.

Serve the fried eggplants garnished with the thyme-honey sauce.

Mustard

Prepare a homemade mustard, and flavour it with the herbs you like!

Ingredients:

7 ounces yellow mustard seeds (you can use also black which is more spicy)
2 ½ tbsp turmeric powder
½ cup olive oil
1 cup apple vinegar
1 cup of water
1 tsp thyme honey
1 tsp ground thyme

How to: Use a coffee grinder or a pestle to turn mustard seeds into powder. Then put all the ingredients in the food processor and process until you get a smooth cream; add more water if needed. Taste to see if you like to add more of something or if it needs any salt and pepper.

Sauces

- **Red sauce with thyme and oregano**

A tasty sauce for all kinds of pasta. You can use it in your pizzas too!

Ingredients:

2 ripe tomatoes (medium to large)
1-2 tbsp tomato paste

1 red onion, finely chopped
3 tbsp olive oil
½ tsp dried thyme
½ tsp dried oregano
¼ tsp brown sugar
Salt and pepper

How to: Wash the tomatoes and cut them into small cubes (you can use a food processor, if you prefer the sauce to be smooth with no pieces.) Warm the oil in a saucepan and add the finely chopped onion. Sauté for 1-2 minutes, add the tomatoes, the tomato paste, the sugar and a little water, depending on how thick you want the sauce. I don't add more than a small cup. Stir an let it simmer for 15-20 minutes; be around to check if it needs more water. Then, add a pinch of salt and pepper, thyme and oregano and stir well. Remove from fire and serve warm with pasta.

As I said before, you can use this sauce on your pizza dough too!

- **Oil-Lemon-Oregano vinaigrette**

The well known Greek "Ladolemono", which means "Oil and Lemon", and it is absolutely yummy with boiled or steamed vegetables, fish, even with fried potatoes.

Ingredients:
1 cup olive oil
The juice of one small lemon
1 tbsp oregano

How to: Mix them all together, using a small electric whisk, until the ingredients unify and the colour gets lighter. It tastes really great!

Oils

Olive oil is not an obsession, it is just the best oil for cooking, and especially if eaten raw in salads (I know, it is quite expensive sometimes). However, you can use any oil you have available, but the result won't have the same taste. Always try to buy organic.

Below I'm giving you two recipes that go with almost every dish, and can be served wonderfully on your lunch or dinner table!

- **Spicy Oil**
  Ingredients:
  2 cups olive oil
  2 red hot peppers, crushed a bit
  1 tsp dried oregano
  1 tbsp dried thyme
  1 fresh oregano twig (optional)
  How to: Put all the ingredients in a clean glass bottle, and keep it in a cool dark place for about ten days. Then, strain with a coffee filter into a clean and dry glass bottle again, add the fresh oregano twig if you like, and it is ready to flavour your dishes!

- **Sea breeze oil**
  Ingredients:
  2 cups of olive oil
  3 slices of lemon
  2 tsp fresh oregano
  1 tsp white peppercorns
  8-10 fresh mint leaves
  How to: Put all the ingredients in a clean glass bottle, and keep it in a cool dark place for about ten days. Then, strain with a coffee filter, and pour into a clean and dry glass bottle. Ready to be served!

Remember that you can try your own combinations, using the herbs, fruits and spices you like the best! Cooking comes out of imagination and good taste!

Vinegars

Recipes for aromatic vinegars

- **White vinegar with thyme and apricots**
  Ingredients:
  3 cups of white grape vinegar
  1 sprig of thyme
  2 apricots (dry or fresh)
  How to: Cut the apricots in half (if you use fresh apricots, use the kernels too.) Pour the vinegar in a bottle with an opening wide enough (to fit the apricot kernels.) Add the apricot halves, the kernels

(optional) and the thyme. Close the cap and keep it in a dark and cool place for 3 weeks before use.

Try this pinkish vinegar with green leaf salads, roasted veggies, as a marinade for mushrooms and vegetables, or whatever tastes good for you!

- **Vinegar with Oregano, Thyme and Honey**
  Ingredients:
  3 cups apple vinegar
  ½ cup thyme honey
  2 tsp dried oregano
  1 tsp dried thyme
  1 fresh thyme twig
  2 garlic cloves, cut in half

How to: In a ceramic pot, simmer all the ingredients (except the fresh thyme), for about 8 minutes. Remove from fire and let it cool down. Use a coffee filter to strain. Put the thyme twig in a clean and pretty glass bottle, pour in the vinegar mixture, and close the cup. Tasty with a decorative look in your kitchen!

Salads

Oregano is the best herb for almost any kind of salad, but there are also a few ideas for thyme too.

- **Beetroot salad with thyme**
  Ingredients:
  1 pound Beetroots
  2 fresh green onions
  1 tsp fresh thyme
  3 tbsp olive oil
  2 tbsp red wine vinegar
  A pinch of brown sugar

How to: Wash and boil, or steam, the beet roots until they get tender. Let them chill a bit and peel. Cut into slices and put them in a salad bowl. Add the chopped fresh onions. Whisk a bit the oil with the vinegar and the sugar, and pour over the beetroot slices. Add the thyme and mix well all together.

- **Oregano summer salad**
  Ingredients:
  2 zucchini, medium size
  2 cucumbers, medium size
  3 tbsp olive oil
  1 tbsp apple vinegar
  1 tbsp fresh or dried oregano
  Salt and pepper

  How to: Wash well the zucchini and the cucumbers. Zucchini can be eaten raw, exactly like cucumbers. However, if you like, you can dip them in hot water for a while, but do not let them become too soft.

  Use a peeler to cut all of them into very thin slices. Put the slices in a salad bowl. Use a fork to whisk the oil with the vinegar, the oregano, the salt and the pepper, and pour the sauce over the salad. Refreshing!

- **Lentil salad with oregano**
  Ingredients:
  1 ½ cup of lentils
  1 bay leaf
  4 tbsp olive oil
  2 tbsp oregano, fresh or dried
  1 tbsp red wine vinegar
  1 sweet red pepper
  2 fresh green onions
  10 black olives without the kernels
  Salt and pepper

  How to: Boil the lentils with the bay leaf, for about 30 minutes. Strain, throw away the bay leaf and put the lentils in a salad bowl. Chop the fresh onions, cut the pepper and the olives into slices. Add them in the salad bowl, along with the oil, the oregano and the vinegar. Season with salt and pepper, and mix well. Enjoy!

Clean and safe household

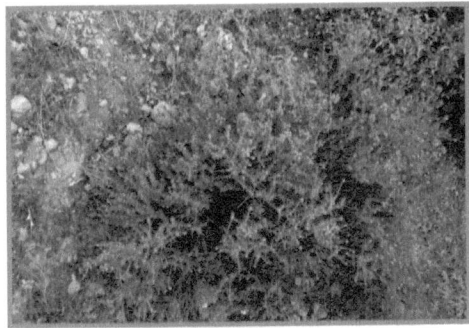

The disinfectant properties of thyme and oregano, are absolutely proper for home cleaning. Plus, their intense scent keeps away all kinds of insects.

Cleaning

Clean your house safely and also save the environment!

- Prepare a mild cleanser for your bathroom and kitchen. In a spray bottle, add 3 cups of distilled water, 9 drops of thyme essential oil and 12 drops of thyme tincture. Very good for for moldiness and fungi. **Notes:** If you don't have essential oil add more tincture, if you don't have tincture add more drops of essential oil. If you want, you can add 1 cup of strained lemon juice.
- Another Eco-friendly cleanser can be made as follows: In a spray bottle, add 2 cups of distilled water, ½ cup baking soda, ½ cup vinegar, 5 drops thyme and 5 drops oregano essential oils. Shake.
- Floor cleaning: in a bucket of water, add 1/4 cup white vinegar, 10 drops of oregano/thyme essential oil or 1/2 cup oregano/thyme tincture.

Repellent

Thyme is an insect repellent plant., while oregano also repels pests in stored goods.

- Plant thyme in a pot, to keep away flies, mosquitoes and other biting insects.
- Diffuse thyme scent with an essential oil warmer or a diffuser.
- Burn some dried thyme as an incense; it is disinfectant too!

- Spread oregano outside doors and windows to repel ants and other insects. I know that bugs don't always use the front door to enter the house, but still, spread it wherever their possible paths are.
- Natural insect repellent for the body: 1 cup aloe gel, 1 tbsp almond oil, 4 drops oregano and 4 drops thyme essential oils. Mix all together and keep it in a small glass jar or bottle.

Basic formulas

Thyme or Oregano oil extract

This is an herb extract in an oil base, which you may use for several purposes as described above.

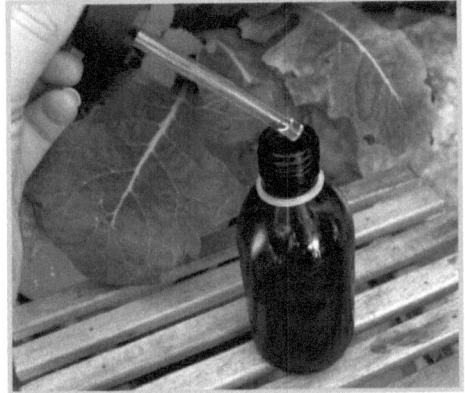

Ingredients:
4Oz almond or olive oil
For thyme extract: 1 handful of thyme leaves and flowers (or 2 whole twigs)
For oregano extract: 1 handful of oregano
How to: Place the thyme or oregano in a small jar with a lid. Add the oil and close well. Shake and let it in a sunny place for about 1 month. Shake the container once a day or at least every other day.

Tips: Remember to take it indoors at night, and place it outdoors again in the morning when the sun comes up.

If the sunlight sees the bottle all day long, 1 month is good enough. Otherwise, if the sunlight lasts only for a few hours each day, keep the sun exposure for 5 weeks or more. Afterwards, strain it and store in a dark glass bottle.

Do not keep oil extracts for much longer than a1 year.

Beeswax salve

This basic recipe of beeswax salve can include several herbs, depending on how and when you want to use it.

Ingredients:
A little less than 1 tbsp organic beeswax (flakes or grated)
5 tbsp olive oil (optionally you can use almond oil)
1 tsp honey (optional)
1 tsp of the herb you choose (shredded)
How to: Use the bain marie method; double boiler. Add the beeswax, the olive oil and the shredded herb in the pot, and stir until

they unify. Add the honey, stir well again and remove from fire. Put the mixture into a sterilized cream jar, and let it cool and solidify. It is ready for use.

Instead of shredded herb, you can add a few drops (5-10) of an essential oil with the properties you want to add to your homemade salve. First, remove the pot from heat, and then add the essential oil.

During winter, when the temperature is low, the cream becomes more solid. You can warm it up a little before use, on the radiator or on the stove while you cook etc.

Notes: Avoid essential oils if you are about to use it on infants. You can store it away from heat and sunlight for about 3 months.

Compress

First prepare an infusion or decoction of the herb. You will need a piece of cotton fabric, big enough to cover the area that suffers. Dip the fabric into the herb infusion, wring and place it on the body. Keep the herb tea warm, and dip again the compress when it gets cold.

Compresses are warm or cold.

- **The warm compress** relaxes tight muscles, increases blood circulation, causes hyperaemia in the affected area, and releases congestion. More blood means more nutrients and oxygen to the injured tissues, resulting in faster healing. The hot compress also reduces pain, muscle spasm, muscle stiffness and joint stiffness.
- **The cold compress** impedes blood flow and circulation. This can alleviate discomfort caused by heat, such as burns, sunburns, infections; it also reduces swelling and pain.

Decoction –Infusion

I'm sure that most of you already know how to prepare an infusion or decoction and what is the difference between them.

Decoction: In a pot, pour 1 ½ cup of water and 1 tsp of dried thyme. Bring to a boil, remove from the fire, cover and let it stay for about 10 minutes. Strain and serve. Add 1 tsp of honey if you like.

Infusion: In a pot, add 1 tsp of dried thyme and pour 1 cup of hot water. Cover and let the herb substances to infuse. You can do it with cool water too, but you have to let it infuse for at least 8 hours.

Poultice (Cataplasm)

Ways to make Poultice: You can use either fresh or dried thyme/oregano.

- **DRIED thyme or oregano:** Use a pestle to crush the dried thyme/oregano leaves. Add as warm water (a few drops) as it takes to make a paste.

Notes: The water shouldn't be too hot. You can also use apple vinegar instead.

Apply this paste directly to the body part that hurts. The herb's therapeutic substances are absorbed as the poultice dries.

Another way to apply, is to fold a layer of this paste within a gauze pad, and place it on the traumatized spot.

- **FRESH thyme/oregano:** Put ½ cup of water and ½ cup herb leaves in a pot and let it simmer for about 2 minutes, until a thick mass is left. Use it as above.

Important: Keep the poultices warm. When you feel that the pain subsides, then the poultice has done its job!

Tincture

Tincture is the alcoholic extract of an herb. (Alcohol 35-90% by volume). Several alcoholic ethanol solutions can be used as well, such as vodka, white rum (alcohol 40-50%) or even strong apple cider vinegar.

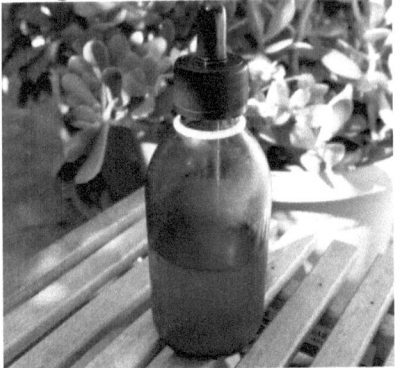

DOSAGE:
A handful of thyme or oregano
1 cup of alcohol
PREPARATION: Do not use metal objects such as knives. Put the leaves in a glass or ceramic jar, with a lid that closes well; no metal parts. Melt the leaves a bit with a ceramic pestle. Pour the alcohol, close the lid and shake slightly.

Place it in a shady place for about one month, shaking once a day or every other day. Thereafter, strain the mixture and store in a dark glass bottle with a dropper, if possible.

The dropper is very useful, since you will be using a few drops of this formulation.

Thyme properties and benefits

"For someone to name all the properties of mint, must know how many fish swim in the Indian Ocean" Naturalist of the 12th century

Antibacterial
Anticonvulsant
Antimicrobial
Antiseptic
Antiviral
Anxiety
Arthritis and rheumatism
Bronchitis
Bruises or swelling
Colds
Depression
Diaphoretic
Diarrhoea
Digestive (fatty foods)
Disinfectant
Epidemics of influenza (preventive antibiotic)
Expectorant
Flu
Gum disease
Hair Loss
Healing of wounds, pimples and burns.
Heart tonic
Insect bites
Inflamed tonsils
Intestinal antiseptic
Leprosy
Lichen
Menstrual pains
Mental clarity
Migraines
Muscle issues
Nerve disturbance

Oral diseases
Physical and mental prostration
Pulmonary infections
Rheumatism
Scabies
Skin disorders
Sore throat
Spasms
Stiff neck
Stimulus
Stomach problems
Tonic
Toothache
Tuberculosis
Whooping cough

Oregano properties and benefits

Allergenic
Anti-altschaimer
Anti-asthmatic
Antibacterial
Antibiotic
Anti-inflammatory
Anti-diuretic
Antimicrobial
Antioxidant
Antiseptic
Atherosclerosis
Bruises and swelling
Calms nervous system
Cold
Diarrhoea
Digestive
Diuretic
Emmenagogue
Expectorant
Flu
Fungicides
Gingivitis
Headache
Intestinal disorders
Lice
Lung cleanser
Menstrual crabs
Muscle and joint pains
Oral inflammations and ulcers
Rheumatism
Spasms
Stiff neck
Throat inflammation
Toothache

Thyme varieties

Below there are some of the most known thyme varieties:

Thymus vulgaris: The common thyme. It has yellow, silver foliage, and it used mostly in cooking. We find it mostly in the western Mediterranean. The cultivated form of wild thyme.

Thymus serpyllum (wild thyme): Got its Latin name by its "serpent-like" form.

Thymus capitatus : (some refer to this species as wild thyme) A small shrub with woody stems which can be found on rocky, mountainous and arid regions of the mainland. *"Thyme, everyone knows it. It is a low shrub in the form of brushwood, covered with many narrow leaves, which have purple flowering tops, and it grows in rocky and infertile soils. When you drink it with salt and vinegar, it expels phlegm from the abdomen. Decoction with honey helps those who have asthma or helminths, it facilitates menstruation and childbirth; it is also diuretic and when is mixed with honey, it helps in expectoration.."* [Dioscorides, "De Materia Medica" 3rd book]

Thymus Atticus (or thyme of Attica): it can be found in various rocky areas of Attica, Achaia, Corinth and Olympus.

T. Zygis: This variety is similar to T.vulgaris, and it is mainly used for the essential oil production.

Thymus striatus: a very common variety in several plains and prairies of Macedonia and Thrace.

T. Citriodorus: Lemon thyme with upright growth and very strong lemon scent.

Varico: A robust variety with upright growth and grey-blue foliage. A great variety of fresh thyme production, and also very resistant to frost conditions.

*The little x means that this specific variety is a hybrid.

Oregano varieties

Origanum vulgare spp. Hirtum or heracleoticum: The most widespread kind of oregano in Greece.

Origanum vulgare spp. vulgare

Origanum vulgare spp viridulum

Coridothymus capitatus: Spanish oregano

Origanum onites: Turkish oregano

Just a couple of quotes before you go...

"Oregano is the spice of life."
Henry J. Tillman

"I know a bank where the wild thyme blows,
Where oxlips and the nodding violet grows,
Quite over-canopied with luscious woodbine,
With sweet musk-roses and with eglantine."
William Shakespeare, A Midsummer Night's Dream

Thank you!

References

1. Evaluation of Efficacy and Tolerability of a Fixed Combination of Dry Extracts of Thyme Herb and Primrose Root in Adults Suffering from Acute Bronchitis with Productive Cough, Editio Cantor Verlag Aulendorf, Bernd Kemmerich

2. Inhibition of enteric parasites by emulsified oil of oregano in vivo, Mark Force, William S. Sparks and Robert A. Ronzio, Article first published online: 11 MAY 2000

3. Thyme: A Herb That Gives You Courage

4. A French microbiologist from Chilly-le-Vignoble in the department of Jura who worked with Louis Pasteur.

5. Oregano could help eradicate MRSA superbug. A natural oil found in oregano could help fight deadly hospital superbug MRSA, early research has indicated, The Telegraph, 6:30AM GMT 25 Nov 2008

6. Naturafoundation.co.uk, monografie, Thymus vulgaris, Phytotherapy

7. Dietary supplementation with two Lamiaceae herbs-(oregano and sage) modulates innate immunity parameters in Lumbricus terrestris, DA Vattem, CE Lester, RC DeLeon, BY Jamison, and V Maitin, US National Library of Medicine National Institutes of Health, Pharmacognosy Res. 2013 Jan-Mar; 5(1): 1–9. doi: 10.4103/0974-8490.105636

8. Parasitology Research, March 2007, Volume 100, Issue 4, pp 783-790, Date: 06 Oct 2006, Effect of oregano (Origanum vulgare L.) and thyme (Thymus vulgaris L.) essential oils on Trypanosoma cruzi (Protozoa: Kinetoplastida) growth and ultrastructure, Giani F. Santoro, Maria das Graças Cardoso, Luiz Gustavo L. Guimarães, Ana Paula S. P. Salgado, Rubem F. S. Menna-Barreto, Maurilio J. Soares

9. New study shows how Oregano oil kills Bacteria, January 11, 2013 By Stephen A. Lawrence

10. Society of General Microbiology, Thyme may be better for acne than prescription creams

11. Phytother Res. 2000 May;14(3):213-4., Inhibition of enteric parasites by emulsified oil of oregano in vivo, Force M1, Sparks WS, Ronzio RA.

Disclaimer

The above information is a sharing of traditional knowledge and experiences for educational and informational purposes. It does not constitute medical diagnosis or medication recommendation. This book is not intended to substitute professional diagnosis and treatment. Also, is not intended to replace any medication you are already taking or the advice of your doctor.

The author and the publishers disclaim any warranties and are not liable for excessive and careless use, for any incidental or consequential damage connected direct or indirectly with the content of this ebook, or the ignoring of the recommendations of your doctor.

The liability, use, misuse, negligence of any recipe, instruction or ideas given in this book is under the total responsibility of the reader.

Author and publisher disclaim also any warranties for the accuracy of the external links content.

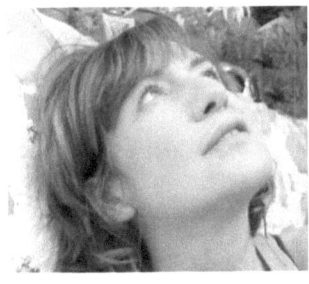

"Hello again!
The third book of the herb series, includes
two quite famous herbs: Thyme and Orega-
no!
I tried to collect the most handy applica-
tions, along with interesting facts and re-
sources.
Thank you for reading!!"

Visit : http://evelinbooks.wordpress.com

for updates, beauty and cooking recipes,
tips and instructions for homemade products,
ideas sharing and lots of colourful images!

www.ingramcontent.com/pod-product-compliance
Lightning Source LLC
Chambersburg PA
CBHW050341290526
45785CB00006B/2592